The Chakras Made Easy

The Chakras Made Easy

Hilary H. Carter

BOOKS

Winchester, UK
Washington, USA

First published by O-Books, 2012
O-Books is an imprint of John Hunt Publishing Ltd., Laurel House, Station Approach,
Alresford, Hants, SO24 9JH, UK
office1@jhpbooks.net
www.johnhuntpublishing.com

For distributor details and how to order please visit the 'Ordering' section on our website.

ISBN: 978 1 78099 515 1

A CIP catalogue record for this book is available from the British Library.

Design: Stuart Davies

Printed in the UK by CPI Antony Rowe

CONTENTS

Introduction

How to Use This Book

My aim in writing this book is to take the mystery out of the chakras and bring them down to the level of everyday life. By healing your chakras you can heal your life. This book will help you to identify and heal chakra imbalance. It can also be used as a useful reference book. However, please note that none of the guidance given in this book is intended to replace medical advice. If you think you are ill see your doctor.

Each of the seven chapters on the seven chakras has the same layout.

LOCATION: This tells you whereabouts in the physical body the chakra is located.

SANSKRIT: This is the traditional name for the chakra. Sanskrit is an ancient Indian language.

ALSO KNOWN AS: These days the chakras are referred to by different names. I use first/second/third and so on in this book but I have listed other commonly used names here.

COLOUR: Each chakra responds to a particular colour. By choosing to use that colour in your everyday life through the use of clothes, curtains, paint, food, cars and so on in the relevant colour, you can help to balance the chakra in question.

NUMBER OF LOTUS PETALS: Each chakra has a certain number of petals.

MANTRA: A mantra is a sound that stimulates the chakra. Chanting the relevant mantra for each chakra helps to balance that particular chakra.

YANTRA: Each chakra has a 'yantra' which is a diagram that corresponds to the chakra. It shows in pictorial form the different number of petals in a chakra. Meditating on the yantras can help to balance the chakras. (See book cover.)

GLAND: Each chakra corresponds loosely to one of the endocrine glands as listed under this heading.

ELEMENT: The first five chakras each belong to one of the five elements. The sixth and seventh chakras are not assigned an element.

BODY: You have seven bodies. (See Chapter 9). Each one is linked to a particular chakra.

NOTE: The musical note associated with the chakra. By humming or listening to this note (or music written in that particular key) you will help the chakra to get into balance.

SOLFEGGIO: This is the exact frequency for each chakra. These frequencies are extremely powerful in balancing chakras. The solfeggio tones can be downloaded from the Internet or you can listen to them on YouTube.

SENSE: The lower five chakras each connect to one of our five senses. Concentrating on the sense in question will help to balance the chakra.

YOGA POSTURE: I give an example of a yoga posture that works strongly on each chakra. Practising the pose will help to balance the chakra. I would advise you to learn yoga postures from a qualified yoga teacher rather than through books or DVDs.

ESSENTIAL OILS: The oils listed under this heading are particularly beneficial in harmonising that particular chakra. You can mix a few drops of the relevant essential oil with a little carrier oil and rub it on your wrists. You could incorporate several of the oils into carrier oil and use it for body massage. You could also put a few drops in your bath or put some on a tissue and carry it with you.

CRYSTALS: I have listed which crystals and gemstones are particularly beneficial in harmonising each chakra. Either wear or carry one of the suggested crystals. You can also lie down and place the crystal directly on to the chakra.

RULES: These are the parts of the physical body that are

affected by each chakra.

PHYSICAL PROBLEMS: Although not exhaustive, I have listed the types of ailments that indicate an imbalance in a particular chakra.

KEY WORDS: A quick summary of the chakra.

WHAT ARE ITS FUNCTIONS? A description of how the chakra will be operating in your life if it is in perfect balance.

AN IMBALANCED CHAKRA: Here I give indications of how an imbalance in each chakra might show itself.

MAJOR IMBALANCE: Under this heading I list more serious imbalances which normally require professional help. If you have a serious imbalance in any chakra do not do any of the exercises in this book without clearing it with your doctor first.

PERSONAL STORIES: I hope that these case histories will help you to understand exactly how the state of your chakras can directly affect your everyday life.

IS MY CHAKRA OUT OF BALANCE? This is an easy checklist to help you to identify your own imbalances. It is meant solely as a guide and by no means is it a fail-safe method of diagnosis. Use the list in combination with your intuition. Although I have quoted numbers to give you an idea of how imbalanced each chakra is, the simple rule is that the higher your score, the more imbalanced the chakra.

HOW CAN I BALANCE THIS CHAKRA? I have listed very practical and simple ways of rebalancing each chakra. Again this list is not exhaustive but is intended to guide you towards your own healing. Healing comes from leaving behind your harmful habits as much as incorporating the positive and helpful activities that are listed here.

AFFIRMATIONS: The affirmations can be spoken out loud as often as you like. You can also write them down on a piece of paper and stick them on your bathroom mirror, your kitchen cupboard or your computer screen to remind you to repeat the affirmations.

HEALING GUIDED MEDITATION: These meditations are very helpful for healing yourself at a deeper level. I suggest you record them on to a CD, phone or iPod, and play them back to yourself when you need them.

Chapter 1

The Chakras – An Overview

A few decades ago very few people had even heard about chakras. Now 'chakra' is quite a commonly understood word. But how many people really understand what chakras are and what they do? In this book I will explain the chakras in a down to earth and easy to follow way. Using that knowledge you will be able to work on healing and balancing your chakras to improve your health and well-being.

My awareness of chakras began over thirty years ago when I was studying energy healing with a tai chi master in London. As well as being able to feel the human energy field, I discovered I could feel the chakras a short distance away from the physical body. My knowledge and experiences of the chakras and the energy system of the body expanded when I began studying to be a yoga teacher with the British Wheel of Yoga. Gradually I became very aware of my own chakras and the fluctuating state they were in day to day. By understanding and healing my own chakras I changed myself and my life for the better. I hope this book will help you to do the same.

What are the chakras?

They are energy centres that connect to the physical body. There are seven main chakras and these are the ones we will be working with in this book. Unless you are clairvoyant you will be unable to see the chakras as they are not physical in nature. Even so, they affect your physical body very strongly. In fact they affect all areas of your life including your emotional, mental and spiritual well-being.

What do they look like?

Chakra (pronounced shack-ruh) means wheel because they look like coloured wheels of energy spinning round. They are funnel shaped, with the narrow part of the funnel near the spine, getting wider the further from the spine they are. The first chakra points downwards from the base of the spine, the seventh chakra points upwards from the top of the head and the remaining five project out from both the front and back of the body. Each chakra spins at a different speed. The first chakra at the base of the spine spins at the slowest speed. The seventh chakra projecting from the top of the head spins the fastest.

What is the purpose of the chakras?

Their purpose is to step down Universal energy so that it is at the right frequency to be utilised by us here on earth in our physical body. Imagine if you plugged an electric shaver into a normal wall socket. It would blow up because too much charge would be going through it. So we use an adaptor. That 'steps down' the flow of energy. That is what the chakras do. In that way you could call the chakras adaptors or transformers.

Where are the chakras?

They are located along the spine. In your physical body, the nervous system runs along the spine and into the brain. Our main energy channel also runs along the spine. It has three channels called IDA (rhymes with leader), PINGALA (ping-gala) and SUSHUMNA (soo-shoom-nuh). The IDA and PINGALA wind to and fro up the SUSHUMNA in the same way that the two snakes wind around the staff in the symbol of the caduceus. The places where the IDA and PINGALA cross are where the chakras are located. These crossing places coincide with the places in the physical body where we have a cluster of nerve plexuses.

Ida Nadi can be compared to the Parasympathetic Nervous system.

Pingala Nadi can be compared to the Sympathetic Nervous System.

What is the sushumna?

The sushumna is a hollow channel along the spinal cord that does not exist in the physical body. It exists in the energy body. This space is the interface between the physical body and non physical bodies. Many people think that yoga is an exercise system for improving the suppleness of the physical body but in fact yoga is a powerful system that helps to clear the sushumna channel, allowing an increased amount of prana/chi/energy to flow through. If energy in the sushumna is flowing freely, then the chakras can spin more easily. The more energy in the sushumna, the faster the chakras can spin, the higher our consciousness.

Think of a basin of water emptying. It spins as it goes down the plug hole in exactly the same way that a chakra spins. However, if your bathroom pipes are clogged up then your basin gets blocked and gunge builds up in the pipe. Then the water cannot spin freely. It becomes stagnant. Some of the water will seep through the gunge and the basin will eventually empty. That is how it is with the chakras. The energy in the chakras can get stuck and 'gungy' and need unblocking.

How do the chakras affect our lives?

Each chakra represents one area of your life.

The First Chakra: The survival instinct. Being grounded and rooted on the earth in your physical body. A sense of security.

The Second Chakra: Relating to the world and the people in it. Finding what brings you pleasure. Sexuality.

The Third Chakra: The ability and drive to complete things. Using your willpower.

The Fourth Chakra: Love, feelings of empathy and compassion.

The Fifth Chakra: Expressing your truth for the benefit of others.

The Sixth Chakra: Intuition. Sixth sense.

The Seventh Chakra: Connecting to spirituality and your higher purpose.

How do chakras get blocked or unbalanced?

We all have chakras and they all spin to some extent. When the chakras are fully functioning they will be in balance and spinning freely. When we have a difficult experience we either unconsciously block the energy flowing through a chakra or the chakra locks open. Either of these will cause an imbalance. A block, a lock or an imbalance are the same thing, resulting in the chakra either under functioning or over functioning.

The chakras can become unbalanced at any time. They are not fixed. They don't get into balance and stay that way forever. They can change moment to moment so it's a constant balancing act, day in and day out. An imbalance in any chakra will affect the entire system. Compare it to a central heating system. If there is a block in one of the radiators the whole system will be affected.

Understanding how the chakras get out of balance is common sense. An injury, a difficult emotional experience, a profound shock or putting too much emphasis on any one part of your life at the expense of another are all the sorts of things that can put one or more of your chakras out of balance. For example, if you sit around all day watching soaps on television, never clean and tidy your home and never go out in nature then your base chakra is likely to be under functioning.

How can we balance our chakras?

To keep (or bring) our chakras into balance then we need to incorporate the needs of all seven chakras into our everyday life. Not only will this be emotionally, physically and spiritually healing, but you will find that your life transforms as you come into balance. Balance your life and your chakras will gradually come into balance. Doing a regular audit of your life under the following headings could be helpful:

Contact with nature / Work and earning a living / Time with family and friends, chilling out, having fun / Health, diet and exercise / Spirituality and meditation / Being creative and expressing yourself / Personal growth and expanding your knowledge / Helping others and voluntary work.

Write under each heading in what way you are satisfying these eight needs. You will clearly see which areas you are neglecting and which you are overemphasizing. You can then make a conscious effort to redress the balance.

Allow your chakras to come into balance rather than striving to balance them. Compare it to trying to relax. If you strive to be relaxed the relaxation will never come as you will be caught in the striving! It's the same with sleep. If you try to sleep you will be kept awake by the act of trying. Sleep cannot be taught. You can put things in place that will encourage sleep to happen, such as dim lighting, a comfortable clean bed, lavender oil on the pillow and soothing music. Then sleep happens of its own accord.

So it is with balancing the chakras. Put into place the activities for balancing the chakras and then allow the balance to happen naturally.

As you read this book, try and remember that imbalance in the chakras is not anybody's 'fault'. If your base chakra was imbalanced by your early childhood experiences or your heart chakra was temporarily put out of balance by the ending of a love affair, then it was all meant to be. A wise person understands that the source of everything they experience is within them. Although accidents, arguments and challenging situations may appear to be coming from other people, at a deeper level you have drawn these events to you in order to grow and evolve.

Chapter 2

The First Chakra

Location: The base of the spine
The Sanskrit name: MULADHARA (pronounced mool-uh-dah-ruh)
Also known as: Base chakra, root chakra, coccyx chakra
The colour related to this chakra: Red
Number of lotus petals: 4
Mantra: Lam (rhymes with lamb)
Yantra: Four lotus petals (see cover)
Gland: Adrenal
Element: Earth
Body: The physical body
Note: C
Solfeggio Frequency: 396 Hz
Sense: Smell
Yoga Posture: Mountain posture
Essential Oils: Patchouli, cypress, myrrh, vetiver
Crystals: Garnet, Obsidian, Ruby, Red Jasper, Haematite, Smoky Quartz
Rules: Bowels, anus, legs and feet, coccyx, lower back, perineum, colon, urethra tubes and bladder, the hips, the male sex organs
Physical Problems related to this chakra include: Infections of the urinary system, poor teeth and/or bones, stiff or painful lower back, sciatica, hip issues, problems in the lower digestive tract, piles and inflammatory bowel disease, skin problems, lack of energy.
Key Words: Survival, stability, acceptance, self-preservation, being grounded, fear and safety

What Are Its Functions?

First and foremost this chakra is about survival. This urge to survive here on planet earth is primal and instinctual. If you fail to survive you die, so the raw drive of this chakra is extremely powerful. This chakra is linked to the adrenal glands and the fight or flight instinct.

It is also about your connection to the earth. If your base chakra is functioning well then you are fully in the physical body and other people describe you as being well grounded. You feel safe, stable and secure within yourself and you are able to manifest and create things in the world. Your life is meaningful and brings you inner contentment and you feel safe and comfortable in your home and neighbourhood.

You respect the needs of your physical body so you don't live on junk food. You exercise and stretch your body without becoming a fitness fanatic. Your home has a sense of organisation rather than disorganisation and you normally manage to keep on top of your paperwork. You manage money well so you won't be in debt. You have a good level of energy and you are able to cope with the challenges of life.

When this chakra is well balanced you feel strong and stable but not rigid. You will be flexible enough to respond to change. Because of your innate trust that the universe will provide for your needs, you are not a worrier. You are quietly confident that whatever happens, everything always turns out okay in the end.

An Imbalanced First Chakra

Imbalance in this chakra is often found in the person who was not cared for in a consistent manner during their early life. You may have been passed from one carer to another, never being able to bond fully with any of them. Your parents may have handled you with anger and carelessness. During the very early years of life we are very dependent on our carers and our ability to communicate our needs and get them met. So, if your cries were not answered, you were not cuddled and shown affectionate touch, and your basic needs were not met then it is quite likely that your first chakra will be out of balance.

Imbalance can happen later in life too. A bad fall that injures the lower part of the spine (in particular damage to the coccyx), a difficult labour (particularly if the perineum is cut or torn during childbirth) or a serious disruption to our established way of life are examples of ways in which this chakra can be imbalanced.

Some people think that the lower chakras are less important than the upper chakras but this is not so. What use is a tree if it has no roots? It would soon blow down in the wind. In the same way, if you do not have a strong, balanced base chakra then you cannot function well in the physical world.

If your base is out of balance you are either going to be too grounded (stuck!) or not fully in the physical body therefore not experiencing life fully.

If your chakra is mildly imbalanced and you have too little emphasis on this chakra (i.e. your roots are flimsy), you have trouble dealing with the necessities of everyday life such as getting your tax return in on time or keeping on top of the housework and gardening. You will be prone to financial difficulties too. You may sometimes have the feeling that you are not in your body, almost as if you are an observer of your own life. You feel out of control and find life a struggle because you lack stability and discipline. You feel insecure, anxious and fearful and find it difficult to cope with the normal demands of everyday life. There will be a sense of chaos and disorganisation rather than order in your life. Your health can suffer due to a poor diet and you are likely to overeat, resulting in sluggishness, obesity and fatigue. Your standards of personal hygiene may be low and there will be a lack of physical flexibility in the body.

On the other hand, if you have too much emphasis on this chakra you can turn into the classic workaholic, putting too much focus on the practical, money-orientated side of life. Others will find you self-centred, controlling and domineering. Sex for you will be about personal gratification rather than it being an exchange of energies involving feelings of love. If this chakra is too strong you will be like the tree that cannot bend in the wind: you become rigid, stuck, immovable and stubborn and have a marked tendency to snap/lose it under stress. An addiction to security and a fear of change will prevent your life from flowing. You are likely to be a hoarder and will have difficulty in giving to others and sharing. The lack of giving comes from a deep-rooted belief that there is not enough in the world to go around. Holding on to possessions and people comes from an inner sense of insecurity.

Major Imbalance

A more seriously imbalanced first chakra produces the bully who rides roughshod over people to the extent of actually physically abusing them. Extreme cases manifest as sexual sadism.

A major imbalance can also show itself as a serious eating disorder such as anorexia nervosa or obesity. Eating is linked to the survival instinct. When we eat too much we trying to ground ourselves. When we eat too little we are avoiding being grounded.

I would suggest that if you have a major imbalance you start your healing journey by seeking counselling or therapy.

Emma's Story

Emma had been in a relationship for a year when she decided to move in with her partner. They found a lovely flat to rent and began to create a home. They bought new furniture and were looking forward to the future when they hoped to be able to buy their own place and start a family. A few months later her boyfriend suddenly and unexpectedly told Emma that the relationship was over and he walked out.

Emma was devastated. What's more, she could not afford all the bills on her own. After a few weeks she fell into arrears with the rent and was eventually evicted by the landlord. She had to arrange for all her belongings to be put into storage and she ended up sleeping on a friend's sofa, living out a suitcase.

Not long afterwards she began to suffer from back pain. She had never suffered from back pain before. She collapsed in the supermarket and was taken to hospital where she was diagnosed with a serious urine infection that had spread to her kidneys.

Emma's Healing

In Emma's case her first chakra had been put out of balance by the sudden actions of her boyfriend. Losing her home left her feeling rootless and ungrounded. She had literally been uprooted.

The first part of Emma's healing involved finding a place to live. She needed a base to ground her. She couldn't afford her own place so she had to rent a room in a shared house. This meant she could take her stuff out of storage, sell what she no longer needed and put her remaining belongings in her room. From this base she now had an address which meant she could apply for jobs. One of her flatmates had a dog so Emma made a point of walking him in the park, getting in touch with nature by doing so.

In the meantime, she made time each day to incorporate other suggested activities under the How Can I Balance My First Chakra? list into her everyday life. She also began to see a counsellor to work through some childhood issues. She learned that she had attracted a boyfriend who rejected her as this is how her father had behaved towards her.

Now Emma has a new well-paid job that she loves and she is saving up to put a deposit on her own place. She holds no resentment to her former partner as she accepts that although she was angry with him for walking out on her, by doing so he had actually triggered her healing journey.

Alan's Story

Alan was a successful sculptor. He had a healthy bank balance and several valuable properties. However, he was not a popular man. He had been married three times and all his wives left him stating the same thing: that he was mean and he was a control freak.

His home was a mess. It was crammed with possessions as he never got rid of anything. He had two children but despite his wealth he hardly ever helped them out financially. He just couldn't give. He clung on to money and possessions. At the age of twenty-two, after a lifetime of putting up with his bullying, his daughter cut him out of her life. At this point Alan's sciatica flared up. He had suffered from a bad back for years but this time it was so bad that he became confined to bed.

Alan's Healing

It was an enlightened doctor who suggested that Alan's sciatica might have a deeper cause. He suggested counselling. Out of desperation and as it was free (Alan would never have spent money on such stuff!) Alan accepted the six sessions offered.

Through counselling he came to the realisation that his father had been a control freak too. Alan's childhood home had been run like clockwork and the arrival of a new baby (Alan) had been a very difficult adjustment for his father to make. Despite his wife's protests, his father had insisted that Alan needed to fit in with his parent's routine. Alan had been fed according to the clock on the wall and not when he was hungry. He was put to bed at 6.30pm each evening and left to cry himself to sleep. If he woke in the night he was again left to cry. His unanswered cries had imbalanced Alan's base chakra.

Alan is incorporating activities from the list below (How Can I Balance My First Chakra?) into his everyday life. He plays the solfeggio frequency every single day and slowly his world is changing. He has started to get rid of some of his possessions and he has written to his daughter asking for forgiveness.

Is My First Chakra Out of Balance?

Your first chakra is either going to be under functioning or over functioning. Read the following statements.

Score 1 if you agree slightly.
Score 2 if you agree.
Score 3 if you agree strongly.

I struggle to make ends meet.
I'm always feeling tired.
I moved house more than three times before the age of seven.
I was disconnected from a parent (through death, adoption or absence) before the age of seven.
I hardly ever spend time in nature.
I hate the colour red and never wear red.
I have injured the base of my spine within the last year.
I feel as if I do not belong to this world.
I am (or recently was) homeless.
People call me a control freak.
I am prone to angry outbursts.
I do not feel safe in my neighbourhood.
I do not trust people.
I am insecure within myself.
I have a very strong sex drive.
My work is definitely the most important thing in my life.
I have a lot of possessions but I need them all.
I have lost my sense of smell.
I struggle to cope with my life.
I have one or more of the physical problems linked with this chakra, listed at the beginning of this chapter (a point for each one).

Add up your score.
Under 5 points: It is in balance.
5–15 points: It's slightly out of balance.
15–20 points: You definitely need to rebalance this chakra.
More than 20 points: Make it a priority to rebalance this chakra.

How Can I Balance My First Chakra?

1. Walk barefoot on the earth or paddle in the sea.
2. Plant and grow your own vegetables or create a beautiful flower garden. Any gardening activities are helpful.
3. Take up a competitive, high energy sport such as rugby or sprinting.
4. Dance outside in bare feet.
5. Bring the colour red into your life.
6. Go into the forest and smell the trees and the plants. Pick up the earth in your hands and smell it. Really connect with the earth through the sense of smell.
7. Spend half an hour a day just concentrating on your sense of smell, wherever you happen to be. You can do this wherever you are.
8. Take up pottery.
9. Hug a tree and really feel its strength and stability. Close your eyes and imagine that you are part of the tree and you have roots that go deep into the earth. Lean against it and absorb some of that deep connection to earth.
10. Practise standing on one leg until you can stay in balance without wobbling.
11. Fill a bowl with warm water and add one or two of the recommended essential oils (see above) and sit with your feet in the water.
12. Learn root lock (mula bandha) from a yoga teacher.
13. Put a handful of salt in your bath.
14. Spend one day consciously accepting every event that occurs to you. Experience how that feels.

15 Treat yourself to a mud wrap spa treatment.
16 Have a reflexology treatment or foot massage.
17 If your house is a mess try to bring a sense of order rather than chaos into your home by clearing up one room at a time. Get rid of excess belongings and buy a filing system to put your paperwork in order.
18 Bring flexibility to your body through yoga, dancing, Pilates, swimming, gymnastics or stretching exercises.
19 Take whatever steps are necessary to make sure you have enough money to live on and a place to live, even if that entails making massive changes in your life.
20 Carry or wear one of the crystals listed at the beginning of this chapter.
21 Bring the colour of this chakra into your life.
22 Chant the mantra for this chakra out loud.
23 Listen to the solfeggio frequency for this chakra.
24 Use the recommended oils for balancing this chakra.

Affirmations

I am supported by the Universe.

I love my body.

I welcome abundance.

All my needs are met.

All is well in my world and I am safe.

Healing Guided Meditation for First Chakra

Stand in bare feet with your feet hip width apart. Your feet are parallel, not turning in nor turning out.

Put your hands on your hips. Close your eyes. Bring your awareness to the breath as it enters and leaves your body. As you exhale make sure that you exhale completely. Allow the in breath to take care of itself. Keep the face soft and relaxed as you breathe.

Now I would like you to imagine that there is a red cord that is attached to the base of your spine. It is bright red, the colour of a ripe tomato, and it's about the thickness of your little finger.

This cord goes down through the ground below you. It goes deeply into the ground.

Breathe in normally and as you breathe out imagine that this red cord is going deeper and deeper into the earth. With each out breath it goes even deeper. Eventually it goes so deep that it reaches the centre of the planet.

Feel that solid connection to the centre of the earth.

Feel that you are rooted to the very core of this planet.

Feel that you are drawing energy from this powerful source.

Now imagine that there is a soft breeze blowing and your body sways gently in the wind. You yield to the wind yet you feel secure in your connection to the earth.

Stand in this place of rootedness for as long as you wish.

When you feel ready, take a deep breath in and blow the breath out forcefully through your mouth, through pursed lips.

Drop your chin to the chest and open your eyes.

Slowly raise your head and bring your feet together.

Smile! You are here on earth in a physical body.

Chapter 3

The Second Chakra

Location: Low down in the abdomen, just above the top of the pubic bone, not far above the base chakra
The Sanskrit name: SVADISTHANA (pronounced svad-is-tarn-uh)
Also known as: Sacral chakra, sexual chakra
The colour related to this chakra: Orange
Number of lotus petals: 6
Mantra: Vam (rhymes with calm)
Yantra: Six lotus petals (see cover)
Gland: Lymph and gonads
Element: Water
Body: Etheric
Note: D (also C#)
Solfeggio Frequency: 417 Hz
Sense: Taste
Yoga Posture: Baddha Konasana (Bound Angle Pose)
Essential Oils: Orange, tangerine, rosemary, juniper
Crystals: Carnelian, Coral, Citrine, Orange Calcite and Amber
Rules: Sexual organs, lower vertebrae, pelvis, the kidneys and bladder, appendix, bladder, hip area, the lymphatic system, all the body fluids
Physical problems related to an imbalance in this chakra include: Problems with the reproductive organs and cervix, infertility, weak bladder or kidneys, ovarian cysts, period problems, prostrate problems, allergies, appendicitis, sexual dysfunction, low back pain (lumbar), sciatica, hip problems, urine infections, loss of appetite for food and/or sex.
Key Words: Sexuality and pleasure, finances, flow, emotions,

creativity, change and movement, addiction

What Are Its Functions?

The first chakra has connected you to the earth. It is through the second chakra that you meet the world and the people who live in it. This chakra is about seeking pleasure and enjoying the sensation of being alive in the physical body with its senses, sexuality, feelings and emotions. What makes you happy and brings you joy? How do you connect and relate to other people? If this chakra is in balance you are able to co-operate with others. You are friendly, warm and compassionate and have a good sense of humour, enjoy being with other people and joining in shared activities. Your life is meaningful and vibrant.

There is an almost childish exuberance in those people who have a perfectly balanced second chakra. They are the people who add that little extra to life, who take the extra step, travel the extra mile. They really live their lives rather than just going through the motions. They enliven situations and add a little bit of magic to the mundane world. They are fully in the physical body and are 100% involved in whatever they are doing. When you are with them you feel that they connect with you and they are fun to be with.

Money and creativity are linked to this chakra, from the creation of a new life through to the creation of your everyday life by the way you choose to spend your time.

The second chakra is also the seat of sensuality and it is from here that you are able to connect with another being with deep intimacy. Although it is commonly referred to as the sexual chakra because of its link with the sex organs, it could more accurately be described as the chakra of intimacy. As this chakra is linked to how you relate to others this chakra needs to be in balance to enable us to relate openly and deeply. You cannot successfully form truly intimate and meaningful relationships if this chakra is out of balance.

The Sanskrit name of this chakra is Svadhisthana. Svad means to sweeten and the more open and balanced this chakra is, the more 'sweetness' there will be in your life.

However, Svadhisthana can also be translated as 'one's own abode'. Sexual abuse is an invasion of your personal 'abode' and usually causes an imbalance in this chakra. By its very nature, sexual abuse is an abuse of intimacy. Victims of sexual abuse often keep silent about the abuse, usually through fear. They can literally 'freeze' this chakra as a form of protection. Sexual abuse at any age imbalances this chakra. This can result in impotence, frigidity or sexual mis-function. If you have experienced sexual abuse, it is likely that this chakra will be out of balance or possibly even 'locked'.

An Imbalanced Second Chakra

Imbalances in the second chakra are common. This chakra is about finding what brings you pleasure. If there is imbalance here then pleasure seeking is either denied or over emphasised. When this chakra is imbalanced intimacy and commitment will be an issue. You may be able to perform sexually but the sex act will be missing the vital element of true, deep, loving connection with another human being. Sex for you becomes the sex act rather than love making and as such it will be a shallow experience. Your relationships tend to be superficial and you use people for your own selfish needs. You will also have a marked tendency towards jealousy which comes from a deep sense of insecurity.

If this chakra is under functioning you are likely to be shy, timid, withdrawn, overly sensitive and to be carrying feelings of guilt and low self-worth. Your life will lack fun, excitement and pleasure. You will find socialising difficult so you withdraw into yourself and avoid contact with others. You fear change and others see you as a rigid person, unwilling to adapt and compromise. You could be frigid through fear of sex.

Conversely, if this chakra is over functioning then no satisfaction is found in pleasure. Instead, you can get caught in the trap of seeking more adrenaline filled experiences. You constantly seek greater and greater thrills in search of that adrenaline hit. Where do you draw the line? When does too much of a good thing become an addiction? (Addictions of all kinds are linked to a second chakra imbalance.) Your emotions are very strong and sex for you can become addictive. You can get attached to people to the point of obsession and when you're in a relationship you soon become emotionally dependent on your partner.

It would be a good idea to attend classes with a well-qualified and experienced yoga teacher whilst working on healing this chakra.

Major Imbalance

At its most extreme imbalance this chakra can create emotionally explosive and manipulative people. Imbalance also manifests as sexual perversions and sexual abuse. Because the relating principle has been imbalanced and the normal relating boundaries are not in place, a major imbalance can produce rapists and the victims or perpetrators of incest. Physical violence (either given or received) and an obsession with sex are common, as are serious addiction issues.

This only happens in the case in very serious imbalances and if you recognise these tendencies within yourself then you need to seek specialist help from a therapist or doctor.

Karen's Story

Karen was only 11 years old when she was sexually assaulted by a paedophile. She was shocked and traumatised by this event. She didn't tell her mother what had happened as she was afraid her mother would be angry. She told nobody.

What she didn't realise was that by keeping silent she had

simply stuffed all her feelings and emotions about the assault. She couldn't own them. She couldn't bring them into consciousness as they were just too difficult for a child of that age to deal with. Unconsciously she thought that by giving this incident no attention, the feelings would go away. What she had actually done was to shut down her second chakra.

From that day onwards her second chakra was locked and her relating ability remained that of an 11 year old. Eight years later she met and married her husband. Theirs was a marriage of neediness and convenience. Their sex life was the sex act with no intimacy. Her husband expected sex at least 5 times a week and if she didn't comply with his demands they always ended up having violent rows. So she usually gave in and allowed him to use her sexually. This regular violation of her body was only possible because of the imbalanced state of her second chakra. A woman with a well-balanced second chakra would not have been able to allow herself to be used in this way.

Karen and her partner tried for a baby but it was discovered that Karen had ovarian cysts which affected her fertility. She was unable to conceive.

Karen's Healing

Karen's healing was a very slow process. She remained married for fifteen years, in a relationship devoid of a close emotional connection and shared intimacy. Then she took up yoga. Gradually, through regular yoga practise and by attending classes with an experienced yoga teacher, the energy slowly began to flow through her second chakra once again.

As this chakra re-balanced through her safe and gentle yoga practise, Karen changed. She began to yearn for the deep intimacy that her unhealed husband could not provide. She had begun to work on her own healing but he had not. She eventually found the courage to end her marriage and almost immediately she met a new man and fell in love. For the first time in her life

Karen experienced what it was like to make love rather than have sex. The connection with her new lover was profound and fulfilling. Although she only stayed with him for two years, this relationship marked a milestone in her life as she knew that she could never again become involved with a man who could not connect with intimacy.

James' Story

James was only seven years old when he was sent off to boarding school. His father had attended the same school and he too had been sent away at this tender age. It was a strict all boys' school and James had been bullied from day one. He no longer played in his parent's beautiful garden in the evenings and at weekends. Instead he sat in the common room doing school work. Nobody cuddled him and there was little time for play. His world became a bleak place that lacked fun, joy and spontaneity. He grew up to become a serious, miserable and money-focussed adult.

James' Healing

For many years James was unaware that he had a problem. He liked sex and, as a handsome, educated and wealthy man, many women were drawn to him. He had no difficulty in finding sexual partners. But he did not respect women. He had a long-term partner but he was not faithful to her. He was always seeking the next sexual thrill. One night he became violent towards his partner when she refused his sexual advances. She begged him to seek help. He refused as he didn't recognise that he had a problem.

Then he was sent on a course through his job. The first few days of this corporate 'bonding' event in Asia involved fasting and having enemas several times a day. (Colon cleansing is an excellent way of releasing old emotions.) It was this experience that triggered the beginning of his healing journey. For the first time in his life he realised that he had never made a close connection with his partner, that he had 'used' her sexually. He also realised that deep down he loved her and he was overcome with remorse at the way he had treated her in the past.

On his return to England he opened up to his partner about his feelings for her. Their relationship changed and they are now living together happily, though both of them realise that they both still have a lot of work to do.

Is My Second Chakra Out of Balance?

Your second chakra is either going to be under functioning or over functioning. Read the following statements.

Score 1 if you agree slightly.
Score 2 if you agree.
Score 3 if you agree strongly.

I am impotent / frigid.
I regularly drink alcohol, smoke cannabis or take other mind-altering drugs.
I go through phases of overeating and have a tendency towards obesity.
I go through phases of under-eating and have a tendency towards anorexia.
I regularly seek out adrenaline filled activities.
My life is empty and lacks fun.
I am shy and blush easily.
I was taught by my parents that sex was 'dirty'.
I have had a restraining order taken out against me (score one point for each one).
I find it difficult to relate to other people.
I am always thinking about sex.
I find it difficult to be assertive.
I have issues around control.
I tend to explode emotionally.
I never (or rarely) buy myself treats.

I never (or rarely) take days off work just to go out and have fun.

I am a jealous person.

I feel unattractive to the opposite sex.

I have been sexually abused and have not received professional help for this.

I have one or more of the physical problems linked with this chakra, listed at the beginning of this chapter (a point for each one).

Add up your score.

Under 5 points: It is in balance.

5–15 points: It's slightly out of balance.

15–20 points: You definitely need to rebalance this chakra.

More than 20 points: Make it a priority to rebalance this chakra.

How Can I Balance My Second Chakra?

1 Wear orange clothes.
2 Eat orange fruit and vegetables (oranges, carrots, swede, squash etc.)
3 Take up yoga.
4 Spend time by water.
5 Run a nice warm bath, put in a few drops of one of the above essential oils and have a soak.
6 Go to Disneyland or a theme park and go on all the rides. Allow yourself to scream on the roller coaster and laugh on the water slide. Just become a child for the day!
7 Spend time helping out in your local pre-school.
8 Buy a CD with the sound of running water in the background and play it whenever possible.
9 Spread a plate with foods that represent different flavours: sweet/bitter/sour. Eat slowly and concentrate 100% on the taste sensations as you do so. You could make this into a game, wearing a blindfold and asking a friend to feed you the foods.
10 Keep a dream diary and learn to interpret your dreams.

11 Book in for a series of massages.
12 Choose a pleasurable activity such as sitting by the sea or kayaking on the river. Be 100% aware during that activity and fully experience the pleasure of what you are doing.
13 You probably know your sun sign in astrology. Find out your moon sign too and read up about it.
14 Swim. If you can't swim, sign up for swimming lessons.
15 Dance. If you can't dance, attend dance classes.
16 Sign up for an inner child workshop.
17 Read up about co-dependency.
18 Drink at least 6 glasses of water a day.
19 Create something (paint a picture/bake a cake/make a model) and give it away.
20 Carry or wear one of the crystals listed at the beginning of this chapter.
21 Bring the colour of this chakra into your life.
22 Chant the mantra for this chakra out loud.
23 Listen to the solfeggio frequency for this chakra.
24 Use the recommended oils for balancing this chakra.

Affirmations

I accept and acknowledge my sexuality.
I am balanced and healthy.
I am willing to receive pleasure in my life.
I move gracefully and easily. My life flows.
Everything is a gift.

Healing Guided Meditation for Second Chakra

Lie down on the bed, the sofa, the floor or anywhere comfortable. Place a slim book low down on your abdomen, partly resting on the pubic bone and partly on the abdomen. Place another one under your body at the base of the spine. Feel these books in contact with your body at the front and the back of your second chakra.

Breathe slowly and deeply. Breathe so that the book on your abdomen rises and falls with your breath. Once your breathing is relaxed and regular and the book is rising and falling, imagine a column of orange light connecting the two books. The orange light shines through your body. This light is cleansing and clearing.

Allow the light to extend down into the earth beneath you and upwards towards the ceiling above. Breathe pure orange light into this part of your abdomen and as you breathe out allow the pure orange light to dissolve anything within your abdomen that is not pure orange light. Any dross just dissolves into the orange light and dissipates harmlessly.

Now imagine that the orange light is orange water and as it flows through your second chakra it cleanses and clears this chakra.

After a few minutes go back to normal breathing. Remove the books and then lie for a few more minutes, enjoying the feeling of a cleansed second chakra.

Chapter 4

The Third Chakra

Location: Just above the navel in the V formed by the rib cage

The Sanskrit name: MANIPURA (pronounced man-i-poora – the 'i' pronounced as in pin)

Also known as: Solar plexus chakra

The colour related to this chakra: Yellow

Number of lotus petals: 10

Mantra: Ram (rhymes with harm)

Yantra: Ten lotus petals (see cover)

Gland: Pancreas

Element: Fire

Note: E

Body: Astral and lower mental

Solfeggio Frequency: 528 Hz

Sense: Sight

Yoga Posture: Boat pose

Essential Oils: lavender, bergamot, rosemary, ylang-ylang

Crystals: Amber, Citrine, Yellow or Gold Calcite, Tiger Eye, Yellow Topaz

Rules: Pancreas, liver, stomach, the digestive system, gallbladder, the diaphragm, spleen, the small intestine, the middle back (behind your navel), the sympathetic nervous system

Physical problems are mostly related to the solar plexus area of the body and include: Poor digestion, liver problems, food allergies, stomach ulcers, gallstones, hypoglycaemia, muscle stiffness, arthritis, diabetes, mid-back pain. Also linked to emotional problems.

Key Words: willpower, action, energy

What Are Its Functions?

This chakra is all about your own personal will. Think of it as the steering wheel in a car. When this chakra is in balance you have both hands on the wheel and you are able to stay on course towards your destination. It's about using your will to decide on which courses of action that you want to take in life and having the personal willpower and self-belief to follow through.

The element is fire and this chakra also relates to emotions and passions. I'm sure you know what it feels like to have butterflies in your tummy when you are nervous. Or that slightly sick feeling in your stomach when you are REALLY nervous. There is also the dread in the pit of your stomach when you have to do something very difficult. All these feelings are directly linked to your solar plexus chakra.

It is fire that gives energy to our personal power. When this chakra is in balance you have the courage to follow your dream and you won't allow the opinions or disapproval of others to sway you from your path. You are in tune with your inner desires and you have a strong sense of personal power. Your life will be a reflection of your will in perfect action. You know the gifts that you have to offer to the world and you will feel a deep sense of fulfilment in your work and in the direction that your life is taking. Quite often (not always) the seeds of your future work were apparent in childhood, such as the pianist who demonstrated an outstanding talent for music at an early age, the school teacher who always took the role of teacher when playing schools, or the engineer who created amazing Lego models.

You have self-respect and healthy boundaries. You enjoy taking on new challenges and you are not afraid to express your feelings and emotions. You feel happy within your own skin and you are able to be spontaneous and expressive. When you say no you mean no and vice versa. You use your willpower in positive ways. You can be discerning without being judgemental.

Not only are you accepting of others, but you accept yourself as you are, without critical judgement. When you are coming from that space, others sense it. This is the chakra that is connected with intuition. I'm sure you know the expression, "I just had a gut feeling." That is you connecting with your gut chakra, the solar plexus.

This chakra is yellow and it is fire. It's your own personal sunshine! When it is glowing with vitality you will give off an aura of positive energy. You will be confident, warm, spontaneous, playful and balanced. You will also be responsible and reliable.

An Imbalanced Third Chakra

An imbalanced third chakra is either going to show itself as the fearful, insecure person or the overbearing, domineering bully. Some people swing between the two extremes. The bully and the victim are simply the opposite ends of the same energy spectrum, depending on whether the chakra is overactive or underactive.

When this chakra is underactive then low self-worth and a lack of confidence will be issues. If your self-worth is low then you do not feel worthy to receive, so you would be the type of person who would charge less than the going rate for your work. Money is condensed energy so by accepting low wages you are actually allowing others to take your energy.

You fear authority figures and others will be able to manipulate you and sway you from your chosen path. "I really wanted to be an artist but my dad wanted me to join the army." Or "I was going to move to the country when I retired but my husband wanted us to stay in the city." Those are the sort of statements that someone with an imbalanced third chakra will be saying.

You will be overly concerned about what other people think of you and what they might say about you behind your back. You are in need of constant reassurance and you don't trust others easily. You're likely to be emotionally and physically cold with a tendency to blame others when things go wrong, thereby playing the role of victim.

You have times when you feel really down and confused and you wonder where your life is heading. You lack a sense of direction and feel as though you are just going through the motions each day. There can be a lot of fear around: fear of other people, fear of emotion, afraid of being alone, fear of your partner going off with someone else and much more. If we go back to the analogy of a steering wheel, your hands are not taking hold of the wheel firmly enough to steer the car so it's going all over the place!

On the other hand, if you have an overactive third chakra you have got your hands so firmly on the steering wheel that you cannot even turn a corner if you need to. Figuratively speaking you will be driving into brick walls. You are likely to try to control everything and everyone around you because you think that unless you take control of a situation, things won't turn out all right. Others will refer to you as a control freak. Excessively ambitious, you can become aggressive and manipulative in your hunger for power. You have an iron will but you don't have discernment to know in which situations you need to use this will. That's why you can end up having arguments over trivial matters so your life can become quite conflict-ridden. It's one thing to use your power to stand up for the rights of the homeless but to use the same amount of energy in preventing someone from eating the piece of cake you have put aside for yourself in the cupboard is a mis-use of energy.

Major Imbalance

If you have a major imbalance then you could develop Obsessive Compulsive Disorder as a way of keeping control of your own little world. You might even need to take medication to control your wildly fluctuating emotions.

The physical effects of a major imbalance are more serious than those of a mild imbalance. Illnesses such as diabetes, clinical depression and gallstones indicate a major imbalance.

Hannah's Story

Hannah's mum suffered from depression. When Hannah was 3 years old her mum walked out, leaving Hannah with her father. There was nothing that Hannah could do to prevent the loss of her mother. As a young and vulnerable child she was powerless to change things.

Hannah's Healing

Hannah was three when her mother left but her diabetes was not diagnosed until the age of eight. Diabetes is related to deeply buried feelings about 'what might have been'. Her childhood had lacked sweetness (see the link with diabetes?) and she had felt unable to cope with what was happening.

There is no doubt that Hannah had a very difficult childhood but her soul had chosen this path. There was nobody to blame, just lessons to learn.

As she grew older she came to the realisation that her mother had been experiencing her own struggles in life when she had walked out and that she had done the best that she could in the circumstances. It was not that she did not love her daughter; she simply did not possess the skills necessary to nurture her. Hannah continued to see her mother and lived with her on and off over the years.

Hannah's diabetes continues to cause concern as she struggles to control this illness that affects so much of her life. She is still young but it could take Hannah more than one lifetime to heal the many issues that she has to deal with regarding her third chakra.

Harry's Story

Harry is a friend of mine. He was brought up in a large family. He had four brothers and two sisters, all very close in age. His father's work meant he was away from home for months at a time and his mother struggled with her large brood. Her coping strategy was to rule her children with a rod of iron to keep them under control. They were never given choices. They were told what to do and when to do it and even how to do it. If they protested, they were physically punished and locked in their room. Harry soon learned to yield to his mother.

As he grew into adulthood it was apparent that his third chakra was under functioning. He regularly suffered from stomach ache with no apparent cause. People walked all over him and he barely protested. He flitted from one job to another, never sure where his direction lay. He met and married a dominant woman who treated him in the same way that his mother had treated him. Harry realised he had a problem with low self-worth. He found it very difficult to look anyone in the eye. When he rowed with his wife he would retreat to the bedroom and close himself away, in the same way that his mother had shut him away in his room during childhood.

Harry's Healing

Harry's healing journey started when a friend asked him if he would commit to being a case study for her Reiki course. As he was unable to say no to anyone or anything, he agreed to be her guinea pig. His commitment turned out to be a blessing in disguise!

The Reiki worked powerfully on his chakras and within a year he was a different man. He was so impressed by the changes he had experienced that he decided to train as a Reiki healer. He is now studying for a counselling diploma to add to his Reiki masters. He has found his path in life.

His wife refused to accept any Reiki treatments or to pursue any other form of healing. As is often the case when one partner begins to heal and the other does not, the marriage did not survive.

Is My Third Chakra Out of Balance?

Read the following statements.

Score 1 if you agree slightly.

Score 2 if you agree.

Score 3 if you agree strongly.

However much I eat I always seem to feel hungry.

I regularly give in to other people's demands.

I don't like my job but I don't know what else to do.

I often say yes to things just because it's easier than saying no and having to put up a fight.

Even though I can drive I always let my partner/friend drive when we go out.

I have never learned to drive.

I earn the minimum wage or I under charge for my work.

I was regularly physically hit as a child.

I find it difficult to look people in the eye.

My partner has hit me/I have hit my partner.

I often suffer from tummy ache or I get a hollow feeling in my belly without an apparent cause.

I feel powerless to change my circumstances.

I frequently feel angry.

I think that deep down I'm afraid of being in control.

I think that deep down I'm afraid of being controlled.

I don't feel good about myself. (Low self-esteem.)

I bite my nails/pull my hair or have other nervous habits.

People tell me I'm a control freak.

I drink or smoke heavily.

I have one or more of the physical problems linked with this chakra, listed at the beginning of this chapter (a point for each one).

Add up your score.

Under 5 points: It is in balance.

5–15 points: It's slightly out of balance.
15–20 points: You definitely need to rebalance this chakra.
More than 20 points: Make it a priority to rebalance this chakra.

How Can I Balance My Third Chakra?

1. Lie down and place one hand just above your belly button and the other one just below, palms facing down and fingers spread. Just concentrate on your breathing. Observe the movement in your hands. They should both be moving as you breathe in and out. If both hands are not moving you need to breathe a bit deeper. Bring the breath into your belly!
2. Eat yellow fruit and vegetables. Also beetroot.
3. Occasionally have a day when you just eat fruit, allowing your digestive system to have a day off.
4. Put a few drops of one of the above essential oils into some carrier oil and use this to massage your tummy with large circular movements. Massage 36 times clockwise and 36 times anti-clockwise with your belly button in the centre of these circles.
5. Find a qualified kundalini yoga teacher and learn how to do the breath of fire.
6. Tone up your abs.
7. Write 'I am worthy to receive' on a piece of paper and stick it on your bathroom mirror.
8. Learn to drive.
9. Take up yoga with a yoga teacher who teaches eye exercises.
10. Have some Reiki treatments or energy healing.
11. Have a bonfire or fit a wood burner or a real fire into your home.
12. Buy some yellow flowers for your home.
13. Wear loose clothing.
14. Treat your liver to a detox.

15 Teach yourself the pelvic tilt exercise.
16 Buy some tinted glasses and spend time looking at the world through different coloured lenses.
17 Buy a relaxing guided meditation CD.
18 Find a good psychotherapist and book in for at least six sessions.
19 Join a gym and get fit.
20 Carry or wear one of the crystals listed at the beginning of this chapter.
21 Bring the colour of this chakra into your life.
22 Chant the mantra for this chakra out loud.
23 Listen to the solfeggio frequency for this chakra.
24 Use the recommended oils for balancing this chakra.

Affirmations

I can do whatever I will to do.

I honour the power within me. I accomplish tasks easily and effortlessly.

In a smooth and healthy way, I release all unresolved emotions.

I claim my personal power now.

Healing Guided Meditation for Third Chakra

Lie or sit somewhere comfortable. You can have gentle music playing in the background if you wish. Your eyes are closed. Keep your eyes closed throughout this meditation.

Take a really deep breath in through your nose and then blow the air out through your mouth, through pursed lips. Do three of these breaths and then sit/lie quietly for a few minutes.

Now imagine that there is a door in front of you. It is bright yellow. Open the door. You find yourself in a bright yellow room with a high yellow ceiling. In the centre of the room is a fire pit with a beautiful log fire burning brightly. You can see a comfortable seat by the fire. Sit on this seat and watch the flames of the fire. Stay in this place for as long as you like.

When you feel ready to leave this room you notice a plate beside your chair. On this plate are offerings: fruit, nuts, rice and chocolate. Take some of the offerings and throw them into the fire. Watch the flames stream upwards as the fire consumes the food. Listen to the crackling of the fire. As you give the offerings to the fire, the fire gives back to you. If you are lacking fire it fills you with pure, raw fire energy. If your inner fire is too great it draws the excess fire from you and burns it away. You leave the room with harmonised fire energy. Thank the fire for this gift of balance and leave the room, knowing that you can return at any time to level your own internal fire.

Chapter 5

The Fourth Chakra

Location: At the breast bone in the front of the body and between the shoulder blades in the back of the body

The Sanskrit name: ANAHATA (pronounced anna-hatta). The name Anahata means unstruck and refers to the Vedic concept of unstruck sound, the sound of the celestial realm.

Also known as: Heart chakra

The colour related to this chakra: Green

Number of lotus petals: 12

Mantra: YAM (rhymes with calm)

Yantra: Twelve lotus petals (see cover)

Gland: Thymus

Element: Air

Body: Higher mental body

Note: F

Solfeggio Frequency: 639 Hz

Sense: Touch

Yoga Posture: Eagle pose and backbends

Essential Oils: Rose, clary sage, sandalwood

Crystals: Rose Quartz, Pink Tourmaline, Emerald, Malachite, Jade, Opal

Rules: The immune system, the heart, the blood and the circulatory system, bronchial tubes and lungs, shoulders and arms, diaphragm, the skin, upper back, ribs, breasts, thymus gland

Physical problems related to this chakra include: Speech impediments such as stuttering, heart disease, asthma, problems with the lungs, high blood pressure, allergies, circulation problems, breast and lung cancer, diseases of the immune system, pain or tension between shoulder blades or thymus

problems.
Key Words: Love, compassion, acceptance

What Are Its Functions?

The first three chakras are more personal in nature than the other four. The fourth chakra is the heart chakra. This is the central chakra of the seven main chakras and you can think of it as a bridge between the three lower chakras and the three higher chakras. It is where the spiritual you meets the physical you. It links the world of matter (the lower three chakras) with the world of spirit (the upper three chakras). The heart chakra is called Anahata, which means 'unstruck' or 'unhurt'. Its name suggests that behind our human experiences of pain and suffering there is a place of wholeness, a place where love and compassion reside. That is our heart chakra.

We often use our heart to express ourselves with sayings such as:

"My heart wasn't in it."
"My heart goes out to you."
"Follow your heart."
"He's heartless."

It will come as no surprise that the heart chakra is about love. Yet there are different kinds of love. The love found here is not just the personal and exclusive love that you might have for a place or a person but unconditional, compassionate love. True love seeks no reward or return for love. Unconditional love does not judge, it just accepts everyone for who they, where they are and what they are. To be able to love unconditionally requires you to love and accept yourself. As you can imagine, finding this kind of love in our world is not easy. That's probably why heart disease is so rampant in our modern world.

People with a balanced heart are authentic. They don't wear a mask or pretend to be someone they are not. What you see is the real person and they are not afraid to reveal that real person because their own self-acceptance makes them immune to the judgements of other people. If someone else doesn't like them, gossips about them, criticises them or laughs at them they see that for what it is. It is the imbalance of the person who is behaving in this way towards them. It is only when we can get to the stage of total self-acceptance that we can feel love and compassion towards everyone, even those who act against us. The more balanced and open this chakra, the more you will be able to feel love and compassion towards yourself and then towards others. Eventually your love will extend to the whole of creation.

As the only chakra that is related to the element of air, this chakra is very closely related to the lungs. Quite simply, if you are not breathing properly (i.e. abdominal breathing) then the chances are that your heart chakra will be silently crying out for more prana/energy.

The heart is the most important organ in the body. If it stops beating we die. Have you ever heard of somebody dying from heart cancer? No, because it is the only organ in the body that does not get cancer.

An Imbalanced Fourth Chakra

An imbalanced heart chakra is either going to be overactive or underactive. In practice that means you will either to be too concerned with the needs of others or under concerned with the needs of others.

If your heart is too open, you put the needs of other people before your own to the extent that you deny your own needs. This can lead to playing the role of a martyr. You'll be prone to excess emotion and manipulating others. You will know if your heart is out of balance if you say things like: "If you do that, I won't love you," or "I will only love you if you…" or "You wouldn't do that if you really loved me."

Constantly drawing on your own resources by constantly giving out to others can leave you drained and stressed. This is where balance needs to come in. It is important to take time for yourself and your own needs. Others can find you demanding and jealous within relationships. Clinginess and co-dependency often indicate excess heart energy.

If your heart is too closed then you find it very difficult to feel real empathy with another person. You won't be able to put yourself in someone else's shoes and feel what they may be feeling. You probably have the ability to harden your heart to others. When you see another human being suffering you might think, "They got themselves into that mess so it's up to them to get out of it." In fact, anyone who can act unkindly to another person is simply displaying a need to be loved. Every unkind act is a call for love.

You'll be wrapped up in yourself, afraid of being rejected or feeling that you not good enough for anybody to love. There will be lots of fears with a closed heart: fear of getting hurt, fear of being rejected or dumped, fear of moving on, fear of making decisions, fear of social situations and fear of relationships. It is often possible to see when the heart is closed as these people hunch their shoulders and physically close the chest area of their body.

The heart can't come truly into balance until you love yourself. That's the key to crossing this 'bridge'. To love yourself requires getting to that place where you can accept all your past wrongs (or what you perceive as being wrong), and with love and compassion you reach that point where you can forgive yourself at a deep level. To do this might require counselling, therapy, Reiki or spiritual healing. Certainly yoga practise will be a good start on your journey to healing the heart.

Major Imbalance

A major imbalance in this chakra can lead to serious heart disease such as a heart attack, a stroke (a stroke is caused by a blood clot – a clot is stagnant energy) or problems with circulation such as angina. All forms of cancer are linked to the heart chakra.

Luke's Story

Luke adored his grandmother. From an early age it was apparent there was a very special bond between them. As they lived in the same town, Luke spent lots of time with her. He would sleep over at her house on weekends and on Sundays they would go to church together.

Suddenly when Luke was 14 years old, his father was promoted at work and he moved the whole family to a city three hundred miles away. A short time later his grandmother died from a heart attack. Luke was on his way home from school with his friends when he was told this news. His father had pulled up in the car and told Luke to go straight home as his grandmother had died that afternoon. Luke said, "Okay," and carried on chatting to his friends, not wanting to lose his cool in front of his peers. In that moment he unconsciously closed down his heart. The shock and the pain of the sudden loss of his grandmother and the way in which news of her death was broken to him were too much for him to handle.

Luke's Healing

Although he was unaware of it, Luke had shut down his heart centre and his relating ability remained stuck at the age of 14. When he met his future wife at the age of 27, emotionally he was still 14. He controlled his wife through manipulation, threatening to leave her if she did not behave as he wanted her to. He found her sexually attractive and he was proud of the fact that she was a successful musician. He loved the image of being married to a popular and admired pianist, but he did not love her as a person. How could he love with a closed heart? It wasn't possible.

When his first child was born by caesarean section, the nurse handed the baby to Luke immediately after delivery. Luke was overwhelmed to be holding this tiny, vulnerable being. A few hours later baby Louis developed breathing problems and was rushed to intensive care. He fought for his life for weeks. Luke spent hours sitting by the incubator willing his son to live. His heart opened to this helpless little baby.

As much as he loved his son, he realised that he did not love his wife. By staying together he was preventing them both from finding true love. He left her. Friends were aghast that he would dare to leave her after she had been through so much, but Luke realised that if he stayed he would be a martyr and would only be staying in the marriage from a sense of duty, not love.

Giles' Story

Cecil adored his only son Giles. His heart was completely open to his only son. Although Cecil lived in sheltered housing for the elderly, Giles visited him every Sunday. One Sunday they had an argument over money and Giles stormed off in a mood. Cecil tried to contact him to resolve their differences but Giles wouldn't even pick up the phone. Two weeks later Cecil had a massive and fatal heart attack.

Giles' Healing

Cecil left Giles all his money in his will and he also left Giles a letter telling him how much he loved him. After the shock of his father's death had passed, Giles was left to deal with intense feelings of guilt and regret. He wished that he could turn back the clock but he couldn't. He is currently receiving professional counselling.

Is My Fourth Chakra Out of Balance?

Read the following statements.

Score 1 if you agree slightly.

Score 2 if you agree.

Score 3 if you agree strongly.

I feel as though nobody loves me.

I don't find it easy to forgive.

People take advantage of my good nature.

I find it hard to feel compassionate towards other people.

I am a jealous person.

I find it difficult to give love/money/time/gifts to other people.

I am shy and lonely.

I am really unhappy in my relationship but I am afraid that if I leave my partner I will be left on my own.

I have a stutter/stammer.

I do nothing to help other people, either within my family or towards humanity.

If I'm honest, there are no (or very few) people that I really like.

I always put myself last.

I am still angry that my parents never told me that they loved me.

I have never told anybody that I love them.

I have feelings of bitterness towards someone.

I am afraid that my partner will leave me for somebody else.

I find it impossible to look myself in the eyes in the mirror and say, "I love you."

I am not physically fit.

I never reveal the real me to other people.

I have one or more of the physical problems linked with this chakra, listed at the beginning of this chapter (a point for each one).

Add up your score.
Under 5 points: It is in balance.
5–15 points: It's slightly out of balance.
15–20 points: You definitely need to rebalance this chakra.
More than 20 points: Make it a priority to rebalance this chakra.

How Can I Balance My Fourth Chakra?

1 Forgive yourself for anything you judge yourself as being guilty of.
2 Forgive anyone you might have judged as being guilty of something.
3 Spend time with babies and young children.
4 Set aside at least an hour a week when you treat yourself as you would treat your best friend.
5 Give an abandoned pet a loving home.
6 Practise the healing meditation (details below) regularly.
7 Buy a heart-shaped mirror and whenever you look in it, say, "I love you."
8 Volunteer in the local homeless hostel.
9 Have some acupuncture to balance your heart meridian.
10 Allow yourself to access deep feelings through a therapy such as psychotherapy or past-life regression.
11 List 5 things that you are grateful to have in your life. Be thankful for these things.
12 Close your eyes. Breathe in through your nose and breathe out through your mouth, allowing the tongue to relax and hang out. Keep the tongue out throughout this exercise. Do this for 11 breaths.
13 Follow your heart…
14 Take up jogging, dancing, swimming or any activity that gets you puffed out.
15 Learn how to breathe properly. (Abdominal breathing.)
16 Massage the area around your physical heart with your right hand, starting at the chest and going all the way

down your left arm. Then repeat with left hand and right arm. (Using massage oil containing one of the above oils would be beneficial.)

17 Book in for a full body massage and really tune into the experience of touch.
18 Accept some healing.
19 Read and/or write poetry.
20 Carry or wear one of the crystals listed at the beginning of this chapter.
21 Bring the colour of this chakra into your life.
22 Chant the mantra for this chakra out loud.
23 Listen to the solfeggio frequency for this chakra.
24 Use the recommended oils for balancing this chakra.

Affirmations

I freely and easily give and receive love.
I am worthy of love.
There is an infinite supply of love.
I forgive, I forgive, I forgive.
I am love.

Healing Guided Meditation for Fourth Chakra

Go and sit in a park or in a café, somewhere where you can see other people. Tap the centre of your chest, just above your heart chakra. (This is where the thymus gland is located.) Tap quite firmly for a couple of minutes and then stop. Feel the energy in this part of your chest. Now, look at each person who walks past you and silently send them love. Imagine that you are energetically connected to each person at the place where you tapped, that there is an invisible cord from your upper heart to their upper heart. See each person as a perfect human being, whatever they look like, whatever their age or appearance and even if they do not look perfect.

Observe what feelings and thoughts arise in you as you do

this.

When you have finished, place your hand firmly on the centre of your chest and silently say, “I love you” to yourself.

Chapter 6

The Fifth Chakra

Location: At the throat in the little indentation
The Sanskrit name: VISHUDDHA (pronounced vish-oo-dah)
Also known as: Throat chakra
The colour related to this chakra: Blue
Number of lotus petals: 16. (The petals contain all the vowels of the Sanskrit language.)
Mantra: Ham (rhymes with harm)
Yantra: Sixteen lotus petals (see cover)
Gland: Thyroid and parathyroid
Element: Ether
Body: Spiritual
Note: G
Solfeggio Frequency: 741 Hz
Sense: Hearing
Yoga Posture: Shoulder stand. Plough.
Essential Oils: Lavender, patchouli
Crystals: Blue Topaz, Lapis Lazuli, Aquamarine, Sapphire, Blue Lace Agate, Blue Tourmaline, Blue Quartz
Rules: Throat, neck, teeth, ears, mouth, jaw, shoulders, arms, nose and thyroid gland
Physical problems related to this chakra include: Thyroid problems, skin irritations, ear infections, sore throat, tonsillitis, laryngitis, mouth ulcers, irritating coughs, gum disease, swollen glands, headaches, teeth grinding, pain in the neck and shoulders.
Key Words: Communication, expression, discipline, speaking one's truth

What Are Its Functions?

This is the first chakra that takes us above the heart chakra. It is the first of the higher three chakras. The fifth chakra is about communication, but not just speaking or writing. It is about speaking your truth and expressing who you really are. Vishuddha means to clarify. When this chakra is in balance our words carry truth and clarity. Most people can chatter on for hours and yet they say nothing. Conversely there are great teachers and poets who speak volumes in a few words.

When the throat chakra is in balance, you trust your inner guidance and you are able to communicate in a clear but non threatening way. You are likely to be a good speaker, an inspired teacher and/or musician. The sense of timing is linked to this chakra. A balanced fifth chakra produces a creative person, who creates through art, drama, singing, music or writing.

Communication is as much about hearing as it is about speaking. Many of us live in noisy environments with the constant distraction of traffic noise, television and background music. How often are you in silence? The mind chatters away inside us. We think nearly all the time. We can only hear the inner voice when the mind is still. The practise of meditation is important in healing this chakra. Sitting in silence and stilling the mind allows us to hear our inner voice.

You probably know somebody with a balanced and fully functioning throat chakra. Without realising the reason, these are the people you seek out for advice when you have a problem. A friend may be able to advise or comfort you but the person you seek will be that person who can view your situation with clarity. Their words carry a deeper truth. Whereas a friend might say, "Poor you. Never mind. I'm sure you'll find another job. Your boss underpaid you anyway," someone viewing your situation with the clarity of a fully functioning throat chakra might say, "You under value yourself by accepting jobs with low pay. Now you are being given an opportunity to change that pattern by finding a better paid job."

An Imbalanced Fifth Chakra

If your fifth chakra is over functioning then you are the person who talks too much. You probably think that what you say is true and that you are always right. Others will perceive you as arrogant. You are not a good listener and you enjoy gossiping about others. You interrupt other people before they have finished talking. You are unable to put any of your opinions succinctly so you're boring to listen to. You might have a particularly loud, grating or unpleasant voice.

If it is under functioning you will be afraid to express yourself, preferring to keep quiet rather than say anything that might upset somebody. Others might perceive you as timid, shy, quiet and fearful. As you feel unable to express your needs, you manipulate people and situations to get what you want. You are likely to choose a partner who will allow you to do the talking for both of you. You have difficulty putting your feelings into words. You probably think, "If I say what I really think people will laugh at me," or "My opinion isn't as good as other people's." You're likely to be tone deaf with a thin, weak voice that lacks power.

Major Imbalance

The throat is where anger is stored and finally let go of. Uncontrollable rage indicates a serious imbalance. If you rage, ask your doctor to refer you for anger management classes. Thyroid problems are common if the imbalance here is major.

Tom's Story

Tom was born with the umbilical cord wrapped twice around his neck. He almost died during birth because of this. As a child he regularly suffered from ulcerated tonsillitis. His father taught him that 'big boys don't cry', and he remembered the feeling of a lump in his throat as he held back tears in order to win his father's approval. That lump was the block consolidating in his chakra. After puberty his regular bouts of tonsillitis started to develop into laryngitis. His laryngitis would last as long as four weeks at a time. He was tone deaf and never sang.

He married young and found himself in an unfulfilling relationship with an older woman. She controlled him and made all the decisions such as where they would live, where they would go on holiday and so on. Tom felt resentful towards her but he was afraid to disagree with his wife in case she left him, so he kept quiet.

Tom's Healing

Tom's healing began when he attended a workshop called, "Healing the Inner Child". It was a group workshop run by a qualified psychotherapist. In one of the exercises the group was taken on a guided meditation back to their childhood. During this meditation Tom had felt that familiar lump in his throat, only this time he was unable to block the tears. The pain was too much to bear. He broke down and began to sob. This was the first time he had cried in public since he was a young child. His mask had finally slipped. He had revealed and released his hidden pain. This incident was the beginning of his healing journey. Gradually he came to understand that his throat problems were the physical symptoms caused by his inability to say what he needed to say. He learned that it was okay to speak his truth. In his particular case he needed to express his anger towards his parents and his wife.

Gradually he learned to express himself but his wife did not want to hear his truth. A couple of years later he left her. Tom has not once had laryngitis since the end of his marriage!

Kate's Story

Kate was a lecturer. Tom was her student. She met him when he was in his last year of teacher training. Tom was ten years younger than her. The physical attraction was strong and they married six months after meeting. Tom moved into her house in London. The marriage had its ups and downs. If Tom did not do what she wanted to do she threw enormous tantrums and screamed and yelled at him until he caved in.

It was towards the end of their marriage when Tom confessed to her that the other students had always dreaded her lectures because she was so boring. He also said that he had always felt controlled by her. Tom had always wanted to emigrate and when he was offered a job in Australia, Kate refused to move. Tom took the job and left his wife.

Kate was devastated when her marriage ended. Her plan had been to have a baby in her late thirties and return to work part time.

Kate's Healing

The breakdown of her marriage was a wake-up call for Kate. Although initially she was shocked to hear the truth that her students found her boring, it led her to realise that she had an issue with communication. She began attending classes in non-violent communication and pinned the following template on her bathroom mirror:

When you ____________ I feel ____________ because I need ______________.

Through regular use of this way of communicating she learned that her anger and her desire to be in control came from a need within her.

She allowed herself to cry. She bought a 'teach yourself to sing' CD and sang along with it in the car on her way to work.

Both Tom and Kate had fifth chakra imbalances and although many people might say that their marriage was a failure because it ended in divorce, the truth is that they were perfect for each other. They mirrored each other's issues and their relationship brought them both to a greater level of self-awareness and healing.

Is My Fifth Chakra Out of Balance?

Read the following statements.

Score 1 if you agree slightly.

Score 2 if you agree.

Score 3 if you agree strongly.

I prefer to keep quiet rather than start an argument.

I was born with the umbilical cord around my neck.

I have difficulty communicating my needs.

If I say what I really want to do he/she will be angry or upset so I'll find another way of getting what I want.

I wish I had a different job.

I scream and rage to try and get my voice heard.

I often have the feeling that something is stuck in my throat and I need to clear it.

I am often told I am critical.

My voice gets strained very easily.

If it wasn't for (*name of person*) I would choose to live in a different town.

I rarely speak up in group situations.

I suffer from depression.

I feel as if other people don't understand me.

I tend to agree with other people rather than argue a point.

I find it hard to express what I am thinking and feeling.

I do things to keep other people happy even if I don't want to do them.

I talk much more than I listen.

I listen much more than I talk.

I lie in situations where it is easier to lie than tell the truth.

I have one or more of the physical problems linked with this chakra, listed at the beginning of this chapter (a point for each one).

Add up your score.
Under 5 points: It is in balance.
5–15 points: It's slightly out of balance.
15–20 points: You definitely need to rebalance this chakra.
More than 20 points: Make it a priority to rebalance this chakra.

How Can I Balance My Fifth Chakra?

1. Take up singing. If you do not feel able to join a choir or sing in front of a teacher, then buy a 'teach yourself to sing' CD and begin singing in the safety of your bedroom! Or play your favourite music in the car and sing along.
2. Practise talking to an empty seat. If there is someone you need to communicate something to, imagine they are sitting on a seat in front of you and tell them (out loud) what it is you need to say.
3. Write an affirmation "IT IS SAFE TO EXPRESS MYSELF" and stick it on the bathroom mirror.
4. Join a yoga group than includes chanting and meditation.
5. Buy a tongue cleaner and use it daily.
6. Stick your tongue out as far as it will go. Hold it out for as long as you can. When you need to take a breath, slowly draw the tongue back in.
7. Lie flat on your back and look up at the blue sky. Feel yourself being bathed in the colour of the sky.
8. Spend a day telling the truth in every single situation you encounter.
9. Have a regular back and shoulder massage to release tight muscles in your upper back.
10. Join a public speaking group.

11 Sit in silence. Start with 15 minutes and gradually increase the time.
12 Express how you are feeling to your friend/partner and ask for feedback. "What did you hear me say? Tell me what you heard me say."
13 If you feel that you do not know who you are or what your truth is, take time away from friends and family to 'find yourself'.
14 Buy a notebook and use it to record your feelings and emotions.
15 If you need to express something to somebody but feel unable to do so, write it in a letter. You can then choose to send it or destroy it.
16 Experience a session in a flotation tank.
17 Enrol in a course in non-violent communication.
18 Explore inner-child communication.
19 Sit or lie somewhere and focus on the sounds around you. Try and hear every single sound within earshot.
20 Carry or wear one of the crystals listed at the beginning of this chapter.
21 Bring the colour of this chakra into your life.
22 Chant the mantra for this chakra out loud.
23 Listen to the solfeggio frequency for this chakra.
24 Use the recommended oils for balancing this chakra.

Affirmations

It's okay to speak my truth.
I express my feelings clearly.
My thoughts and opinions are valuable.
I am a creative person and it is safe to create.

Healing Guided Meditation for Fifth Chakra

Sit comfortably on a chair with the spine upright. Close your eyes. Observe the feelings and sensations in your head, throat and upper body.

Then chant OM (AUM) 3 times. Make each AUM nice and long.

(To chant AUM you start with the mouth open and say AH – it rhymes with car. As your mouth starts to close the AH changes to UH – rhymes with ugh. When your mouth closes the sound changes to MMMMmmmmmmm.)

Now observe the feelings and sensations in your head, throat and upper body. Keep your face relaxed whilst you observe. Be aware of any subtle changes.

Repeat up to eleven times. (33 AUM's in total.)

When you have finished omming place your feet firmly on the floor. Feel them in close contact with the ground. Breathe in through your nose and as you breathe out mentally send the energy down into the ground through your feet. Do this three times.

Chapter 7

The Sixth Chakra

Location: On the centre of the forehead slightly above the level of the eyebrows
The Sanskrit name: AJNA (pronounced aj-nuh)
Also known as: Third eye, Brow chakra
The colour related to this chakra: Indigo
Number of lotus petals: 2
Mantra: Om (Aum)
Yantra 2 lotus petals (see cover)
Gland: Pituitary
Element: None
Body: Soul
Note: A
Solfeggio Frequency: 852 Hz
Sense: Clairvoyance
Yoga Posture: Alternate nostril breathing
Essential Oils: Juniper, peppermint, rosemary, geranium
Crystals: Sapphire, Quartz Crystal, Amethyst, Sodalite, Azurite
Rules: The brain, nervous system, eyes, ears, nose, sinuses, forehead, temples
Physical problems related to this chakra include: Glaucoma, headaches, migraines, visual disturbances, catarrh, mental illness, sinus problems, ear problems, issues with the lymphatic and endocrine system, hormonal imbalances, insomnia, facial nerve problems, nightmares, brain tumours, neurological disturbances, seizures.
Key Words: Intuition, imagination

What Are Its Functions?

This is the sixth chakra and it relates to sixth sense. Sometimes known as the third eye, this chakra, when balanced and open, sees the unseen worlds as opposed to the physical eyes which see the physical world. When this chakra is functioning well you are able to tune into your Higher Self, the spiritual part of you. You are so strongly intuitive that you just know things without having to be told. You can see your life path clearly and are able to think and plan ahead to allow your life purpose to manifest. You're not attached to the material universe as you know that it is transitory. You have no fear of death as you understand that death is simply a transition.

A well-balanced sixth chakra guides you towards making decisions that are good for your soul. Decisions that are made using only the mind and not the intuition can lead you away from your spirituality.

You may experience telepathy, clairaudience, visions, déjà vu, precognition and other psychic phenomena. Memories of past lives can spontaneously arise.

An Imbalanced Sixth Chakra

If your sixth chakra is under functioning you completely block anything that cannot be seen and felt. To you, reason and intellectual argument are the only valid ones and you only accept logic as truth. You block anything that cannot be scientifically proven and in doing so you block your spirituality. You probably don't remember your dreams or you might even say that you don't dream at all. You have difficulty seeing where you are heading in life. You lack imagination. You are afraid of success and feel as if you have nothing of value to contribute to the world.

If it is imbalanced the other way so that it is over functioning you can lose sense of reality. Your imagination can become overactive to the point of being delusional. You could suffer from regular nightmares and headaches. You may have difficulty concentrating which leads to muddled thinking, and this will be reflected in your life as a sense of disorder. You are likely to have great difficulty in planning ahead. You might have difficulty discerning between imagination and reality. Others might accuse you of living in a dream world.

Obsessiveness in all of its forms is linked to this chakra, the classic example being the religious fanatic who tries to force their beliefs on other people.

Major Imbalance

Major imbalances in the sixth chakra can lead to schizophrenia and other serious mental illnesses. These conditions need professional help.

Ian's Story

Ian grew up in a family where business achievements were seen as proof of a successful man. Ian was a Pisces, a sensitive and psychic child who spent his early years playing with an imaginary playmate. His parents sent him to a renowned fee-paying school to ensure that he made it to a top university to study law as his father had done. Ian loved music and dreamed of becoming a pianist or a guitarist. He was slow to learn at school and had difficulty concentrating. At the age of 11 he was diagnosed with myopia and started wearing glasses. From the age of 12 onwards his evenings were spent at the dining room table with an after-school tutor, cramming for exams. Despite the extra tuition he failed to get into university so his father helped to set him up in business as an estate agent.

In his late 20s Ian began suffering from debilitating migraines. By the time he was approaching his 40th birthday his migraines had become so bad that he regularly ended up spending days in bed. As he was self-employed, his business began to suffer and in the end he went bankrupt. He lost his home and his wife left him, calling him a failure. He then suffered a mental breakdown and was admitted into a psychiatric hospital.

Ian's Healing

There is no denying that Ian had a massive mid-life crisis. It was only when he looked back at this crisis that he realised it had been a blessing in disguise. He realised that for 40 years he had been living a lie. He had not been true to himself. He had ignored his inner voice, his intuition. The breakdown was a breakthrough. Although at first he was very angry to think that his life had been directed by his parents, through counselling he gradually came to understand that at a soul level he had chosen this path and that he was responsible for the life he had created. Only he could change his life.

He is currently involved in establishing a community-owned musician's café. He has visions of incorporating a recording studio and a live stage set-up where musicians young and old can congregate, arrange to meet, make contact with each other and perform. Ian hopes to join them on stage at some time in the future as he is currently learning to play the piano. He is showing a natural talent as a jazz pianist.

Sue's Story

Sue's daughter Terri was 17 years old. She was going out with a boyfriend who had a motorbike. Terri told her parents she was going on a camping holiday with him. Sue had a strong feeling of danger and begged her not to go. Terri's father told Sue that she needed to "let go of the reins", and allow her daughter to grow up. In the end Sue relented, Terri went on holiday and was involved in an accident in which she lost her leg below the knee. Sue was distraught and blamed herself for not trusting her intuition enough to stop her daughter from going. She began having dreadful nightmares and slowly slipped into clinical depression.

Sue's Healing

It was her doctor who suggested to Sue that she take up yoga to calm her nerves. Through yoga practise and living the yoga teachings, Sue gradually came to realise that Terri's accident was not her fault. She was not to blame. Terri was on her own journey of life and losing her leg was part of her path. Now Terri has forgiven herself and she takes notice of her intuition and allows it to guide her in her decision making.

Is My Sixth Chakra Out of Balance?

Read the following statements.

Score 1 if you agree slightly.
Score 2 if you agree.
Score 3 if you agree strongly.

I don't really know what spirituality is.
I am afraid of death.
I am highly impressionable.
I find it really difficult to focus or concentrate on something for long periods of time.
I never plan ahead.
If it wasn't for (*name of person*) I would be living my life in a different way.
I regularly have nightmares.
I feel as if my life is stuck.
I have very poor co-ordination.
Intuition is a load of nonsense.
My life is going nowhere. I just have to make an effort to get through each day.
I rarely (or never) dream.
A wise person only uses their head to make decisions.
I am obsessive.
Science is my God.
The physical universe is the only universe that exists.

Mystics, psychics and people who channel messages from other dimensions are delusional.
I am afraid of what other people will think of me if I do what I really want to do.
When I look at other people's lives, they all seem so much more together than mine.
I have one or more of the physical problems linked with this chakra, listed at the beginning of this chapter (a point for each one).

Add up your score.
Under 5 points: It is in balance.
5–15 points: It's slightly out of balance.
15–20 points: You definitely need to rebalance this chakra.
More than 20 points: Make it a priority to rebalance this chakra.

How Can I Balance My Sixth Chakra?

1. Research visual stimulation.
2. Play memory games with cards such as snap or patience.
3. Start keeping a dream diary.
4. Learn eye exercises from a yoga teacher.
5. Take up meditation.
6. Find a Body Talk therapist and learn the reciprocals technique.
7. Have some craniosacral therapy sessions.
8. Spend time in nature.
9. Try guided meditation. You can either download some meditations online, use a CD or find a yoga teacher who incorporates guided meditation into their classes.
10. Join an art group, learn how to draw mandalas and explore your artistic side.
11. Buy an illustrated book of optical illusions and keep it on your coffee table, using it whenever you have some spare

moments.

12 Buy a light that changes colour and sit and watch it.
13 Each evening reflect on the day and make a note of the three most beautiful things you saw that day. It could be a work of art, a flower or an act of kindness.
14 Listen to classical music, especially in the key of A.
15 Rub your palms vigorously together until they are hot. Place them over your open eyes. Feel your eyes drinking in the warmth. When you can no longer feel any heat, close your eyes and remove your hands. Sit quietly for a few moments.
16 Place your right palm on your right temple and your left palm on your left temple, allowing your fingers to point towards the back of your head. Press gently but firmly. Stay for a few minutes then release your hands and sit quietly for at least 5 minutes.
17 When the phone rings practise 'sensing' who is calling before you pick up.
18 Have a few sessions with a past-life regression therapist.
19 Have a Shirodhara treatment (oil drip therapy).
20 Carry or wear one of the crystals listed at the beginning of this chapter.
21 Bring the colour of this chakra into your life.
22 Chant the mantra for this chakra out loud.
23 Listen to the solfeggio frequency for this chakra.
24 Use the recommended oils for balancing this chakra.

Affirmations

My intuition is strong. I trust my intuition.
I can see clearly.
I trust my inner wisdom.

Healing Guided Meditation for Sixth Chakra

Sit or lie in a comfortable upright position with your eyes closed.

Place your index finger on your third eye, in the centre of the point just above your eyebrows. Gently rub this point up and down, not side to side. Keep your inner gaze on the point where you are rubbing. After a couple of minutes stop rubbing and rest your hands on your knees or by your side. The eyes remain closed as you keep the inner gaze on this third eye point. Observe any sensations you experience. Breathe softly through the nose as you observe. If thoughts arise in the mind allow them to drift away again and bring your focus back to the forehead. Stay in this position for as long as you like.

When you are ready to finish, rub the palms of your hands together vigorously to create heat and place the hot palms on your feet until the heat dissipates.

Chapter 8

The Seventh Chakra

Location: At the top of the head. Just as the base chakra forms a downward funnel connecting us to the earth, the crown chakra forms a funnel of energy opening upwards.
The Sanskrit name is SAHASRARA (pronounce sa-has-rah-ruh)
Also known as: The crown chakra, thousand-petalled lotus
The colour related to this chakra: Violet (sometimes with white or gold edges)
Number of lotus petals: 1000
Mantra: none
Yantra: A lotus with a thousand petals (see cover)
Glands: Pineal
Element: None
Body: Nirvanic
Note: B
Solfeggio Frequency: 963 Hz
Sense: None
Yoga Posture: Headstand
Essential Oils: Lotus, ylang-ylang, jasmine, frankincense
Crystals: Blue Sapphire, Amethyst, Diamonds, Clear Quartz, Selenite
Rules: The muscular and skeletal system, skin, central nervous system, the brain and the circulatory system
Physical problems related to this chakra include: Epilepsy, headaches and migraines, hysteria, stress-related disorders (highly strung), psychosis, nervous tension, sleep disorders, coma, brain tumours, short-term memory loss, chronic exhaustion (M.E.), oversensitivity to outside stimulus, depression arising from feelings of emptiness.

Key Words: Knowing, wisdom, self-mastery

What Are Its Functions?

This chakra is of the finest energy and it is the highest of the seven main chakras. It is connected to your spiritual self. It is through this chakra that you are able to enter the highest states of consciousness. When it is functioning to its maximum the seventh chakra brings the right and left hemispheres of your brain into balance. Once it is fully awakened and in perfect balance, you become an instrument of love in action. It is through the crown that the soul comes into the body and it leaves from the crown at death. In this high state of consciousness you feel a spiritual connection with everyone and everything. You become a wise and intelligent human being. You are discerning but non-judgemental and you have the ability to analyse and assimilate information.

In truth you are an instrument of light. Getting all seven chakras into balance and spinning to their maximum is the aim. Once you have succeeded in doing that you can then be that instrument of light. Think of it like a light bulb. Imagine you are a brilliant 100 watt bulb. If the glass of your bulb is cloudy or dirty then despite the fact that you are 100 watts, you won't be giving out much light. The more you clean your bulb, the more light can shine through. How do you get that bulb clean? The best way to ensure a safe and balanced opening of this chakra is by working on the other six chakras. Then the crown will open of its own accord when it is ready.

Once you have become a fully functioning light bulb (!) you can carry the light out into the world, helping your fellow human beings, animals and the environment. You will have moved beyond fear and you will have the ability to take huge leaps of faith. Your intuition will be deep and powerful. You will be courageous, inspired and full of the joy that comes from living a life beyond the ego. You'll know when you're at that stage because by then you no longer think of yourself. All you'll be concerned about is asking, "How can I be of help?" or "How can I be used to help others?"

This is the chakra of total surrender of the ego. However, not only does it need to be in balance within itself but it is vitally important that an open seventh chakra is balanced by a perfectly harmonised first chakra. The more energy that flows through this chakra, the deeper the surrender to Divine will.

An Imbalanced Seventh Chakra

If your seventh chakra is under functioning, you feel as if your life lacks joy. Decision making can be a real issue for you. You are prone to apathy and you're cynical about other people's belief systems. You are likely to hold rigid belief systems which can lead you to forcing your beliefs down other people's throats. Others will find you domineering.

If it's over functioning you will have a tendency to over intellectualise. Your life will lack purpose and meaning. Lacking depth, you will try and fill your life with transient pleasures and acquisitions such as material gain, social status and various pleasurable activities.

Major Imbalance

A major imbalance can lead to a complete disassociation from the body, leading to psychotic episodes. This level of imbalance requires professional help.

Bruce's Story

Bruce was travelling in Nepal when he took drugs. He had a mystical experience in the mountains and found himself talking to beings of light. He had visions of angels and demons. A couple of weeks later he returned to his home in England. He began to suffer from acute paranoia and he ended up being sectioned under the Mental Health Act. He was given electric shock treatment in the psychiatric hospital.

Bruce's Healing

If it wasn't for the fact that his brother was a doctor, Bruce might still be in that hospital. His brother managed to get him released and took him to his own home to care for him. What Bruce needed more than anything was a stable, safe, secure place where he could start working on strengthening his first chakra. The drugs had blown his seventh chakra wide open before it was ready. He completely lost touch with the reality of the physical plane of existence. The imbalance between his first and seventh chakras was immense. Gradually, with the help of his brother, Bruce came 'back down to earth' and now he has a responsible job working with troubled teenagers. He still has the memory of his visions in Nepal and he now has a strong belief in other realms of being, though he is not pursuing a mystical path in this life. Nor does he ever touch drugs...

Harriet's Story

Harriet was a highly intelligent girl. By the age of eighteen she had read all the classics and had come to the conclusion that there was no purpose to life. She leaned heavily towards existentialism and as she thought she only had one life she was going to make it count. She decided to become an artist. All her time, money and energy were focussed on her goal: to become a successful, wealthy and famous painter.

In her late thirties she became pregnant. It was unplanned. She was in a huge dilemma because she didn't want to abort the baby but she didn't want a child. It would interfere with her work. Reluctantly she decided to give birth to the baby. She employed an au pair to care for it. At the age of nine weeks her daughter died from a cot death. Harriet was riddled with guilt. She had told everyone that she really didn't want the baby and now the baby had gone. Her mind couldn't process that sequence of events. She was so traumatised that she could no longer paint and she slid into depression.

Harriet's Healing

The death of her daughter was Harriet's awakening. Her whole life plan had been based on an intellectual understanding of the world. When she lost her baby her intellect could not explain this event. Her grief was immense. She called out to the Universe for answers. "I'll do anything you want," she screamed. "Just tell me why this happened and what it all means."

A short time later she was invited to a Buddhist retreat centre. This sparked her interest in Buddhist philosophy. Her seventh chakra gradually came into balance through studying and living the teachings of Buddha.

Although still a painter, her work now comes from the spiritual part of her. Instead of being an expression of her keen intellect, her paintings reflect her balanced seventh chakra. Her goal now is not to be rich and famous through her paintings, but to bring pleasure to others through her work. She now sees herself as an instrument of Divine Intelligence, creating inspired and inspiring paintings for the upliftment of Humanity.

Is My Seventh Chakra Out of Balance?

Read the following statements.

Score 1 point if you agree slightly.
Score 2 points if you agree.
Score 3 points if you agree strongly.

I feel alone and disconnected from life.
I was brought up in a family with no religious or spiritual beliefs.
I do not believe in a God or Divine energy.
The spiritual side of me feels empty.
Prayer is a waste of time.
If humans on the other side of the world are starving it's no

concern of mine.

I'm really indecisive.

Intellectual arguments are more valid than mystic visions in understanding the meaning of life.

There is nothing to learn from difficult life experiences.

Life treats me badly.

My religion/belief system is the only valid one.

The physical world is the only world that exists.

I believe that we are born and then we die, end of story.

The most important thing in my life is to become wealthy.

I often feel spaced out, as if I'm not fully in my body.

Coincidences have no meaning.

My life has no meaning.

I don't know what I want in life.

I just want to spend my life having fun.

I have one or more of the physical problems linked with this chakra, listed at the beginning of this chapter (a point for each one).

Add up your score.

Under 5 points: Your chakra is in balance.

5–10 points: Your chakra is slightly out of balance.

10–15 points: Your chakra needs balancing.

15–20 points: Make it a priority to balance this chakra.

How Can I Balance My Seventh Chakra?

1 Place one of the above crystals in a glass of spring water and put it in a place where the sun shines through the glass. Allow the room to fill with this light crystal energy.

2 Wear an orgone generator.

3 Sleep with an orgone generator placed behind or above the head of your bed.

4 Learn to meditate.

5 Learn to stand on your head (Sirsasana pose) under the

direction of a qualified yoga teacher.

6 Work on balancing your other chakras and allow the crown to open of its own accord.

7 Do a course on the major world religions or a philosophy course.

8 Imagine you only had five years to live. Set five goals you would like to achieve before that time is up.

9 Take up a spiritual discipline such as tai chi, meditation or chanting.

10 Attend classes in Japanese Tea Ceremonies.

11 Go for a walk and count your steps as you walk. If you lose count or forget to count go back to number one.

12 Learn the tense and release method of relaxation.

13 Breathe in through your nose and blow the air out through your mouth, pursing your lips as you do so. Repeat 11 times.

14 Have an Indian head massage.

15 Find somewhere silent (old churches are good for this!) and simply sit and listen to the silence.

16 Hang one of the recommended crystals for this chakra above your head. Sit quietly beneath it.

17 Using good quality incense or dried sage leaves, surround your body with the smoke to cleanse your aura.

18 Have a Reiki healing session.

19 Buy a tuning fork (note B) and strike it. Follow the sound until you cannot hear it any more. Have a moment of silence then strike it again. Strike it a total of 11 times.

20 Carry or wear one of the crystals listed at the beginning of this chapter.

21 Bring the colour of this chakra into your life.

22 Reflect on the phrase: "I am that I am".

23 Listen to the solfeggio frequency for this chakra.

24 Use the recommended oils for balancing this chakra.

Affirmations

I am guided by my own inner wisdom.
I am a Divine being in a physical body.
Everybody I meet is my teacher.
Everything I experience is good for me.
I trust life.

Healing Guided Meditation for Seventh Chakra

Choose a peaceful and comfortable place to sit. Sit with the spine upright and have your feet on the floor. Close your eyes. Press your right hand gently on the top of your head and then remove it. Rest your hands comfortably on your lap or on the arms of your chair. Feel the imprint of your hand that has been left on the crown of your head. Now do nothing except breathe. Keep a soft smile on your face as you breathe. Although your eyes are closed, keep your inner gaze towards your crown.

When you are ready, press the top of your head gently with your left hand and then remove it. Feel the imprint of your hand again. Breathe. Keep the inner gaze upwards.

When you are ready to finish, bring your hands together in prayer pose in front of your heart centre. Drop your head to your chest. Raise your head. Feel your feet planted firmly on the floor. Smile. You are a Divine being in a physical body.

Chapter 9

The Seven Bodies

Human beings are not just physical bodies. According to the teachings of yoga, we have seven bodies, one physical and six non physical. These six unseen bodies are known as the energy bodies. Although the energy bodies are not visible to most of us, that doesn't mean they don't exist. We can't see electricity either but we know it exists.

The six non physical bodies are not separate from the physical body. All seven bodies are interconnected. They permeate each other. The health of any of the seven bodies contributes towards the overall physical, mental, emotional and spiritual well-being of a person.

Think of your physical body and how it operates. What you eat affects it. If you eat too much, you get fat. If you eat too little, you become thin. A healthy balanced diet gives you glowing skin and silky hair. If you eat loads of junk food your skin becomes spotty, your hair dull and your body bloated and podgy.

The energy bodies are affected in a very similar way to the physical body. They are affected by all aspects of our lifestyle. The energy that feeds our unseen bodies comes from without and within. What you think, feel, eat, say, read, hear and experience all influence your energy bodies. Even the people you hang out with and the places you choose to spend time in affects these bodies.

The physical body is fed by food whereas the energy bodies are fed by an energy called prana or chi. The health of the energy bodies depends on the amount and the quality of energy that is flowing through them. The seven bodies are:

1: Physical

This is the body you are familiar with, the physical body, the one that you live in. This is the densest of the bodies. The physical body does not reincarnate. It is linked to the first chakra.

2: Etheric

The etheric body is linked to the second chakra. It is the blueprint for our physical body. The etheric body is slightly larger than the physical. It is very similar to the physical body in that it has internal organs, a torso, limbs and a head. In appearance it looks like very fine strands of blue or grey light formed to resemble the physical body. It is made of vibrating energy. It underlies the physical and it is semi-transparent. When someone loses a body part such as a leg, they can still experience pain in the missing leg. That's because the leg still exists in the etheric body. The etheric body does not reincarnate.

3: Astral

The astral body is linked to the third chakra. Some people refer to this as the emotional body. It has a resemblance to your physical body but it's less dense. It is like transparent vapour. It is much more fluid than the physical body, almost ghost-like. It is formed of different colours and these colours are constantly changing and fluctuating according to how you are feeling at any given time. For example, if you lose your temper the astral body will be flashed with red until your anger subsides. Emotional experiences are stored in the astral body. The astral body does not normally reincarnate. It can exist for centuries after the death of its physical counterpart. Ghosts are astral in nature. When you dream you travel in your astral body. If you become conscious whilst dreaming you are astral travelling.

4: Lower and Higher Mental Bodies

The mental body is in two parts, the lower and the higher. The lower mental body links to the third chakra and the higher mental body to the fourth chakra.

The lower mental body is the mind of our everyday thinking. It is the mind that we use to reason, to form mental arguments, to create thought forms and to memorise things. The lower mental body forms part of your personality.

In the physical body you are what you eat. In the mental body you are what you THINK. If you are always thinking negative thoughts then eventually those thoughts can permeate through into the physical body. This fact is recognised in books such as Louise Hay's *Heal Your Body* book. That is why changing our thoughts can change our health. As it is part of your personality the lower mental body does not reincarnate. It is only used for a single life.

The higher mental body does reincarnate. You take it with you life after life. As we develop spiritually we raise our consciousness and it is through the higher mind that we can contact the One Mind. That's the mind that contains all information. We contact the higher mind when we are deep in meditation. Have you ever noticed that quite often after meditation you get a 'eureka' moment? Or you have moments of just knowing something but you can't explain how you know? That's because you have opened up to your higher mental body and dipped into the vast ocean of knowingness. The higher mental body is spiritual in nature, and because of this fact it is not concerned with the little self, the ego. Once you are able to keep your consciousness in the higher mental body the ego loses its grip.

5: Spiritual Body

The physical, etheric, astral and lower mental bodies belong to the lower planes of existence. They do not reincarnate. The higher mental, spiritual, soul and nirvanic bodies are more spiritual in nature. They do reincarnate. The spiritual body is the essence of you and contains all the qualities, talents and spiritual attainments you have developed over your many lives. It links you to the collective consciousness of the planet and your soul group. It is linked to the fifth chakra and it forms part of your Higher Self. This contains memory of all the lives you have lived and all that you have learned and experienced in those lives. It even knows about all future life personalities because it can function beyond time and space.

6: Soul Body

The soul body holds the part of you that is of God. It is linked to the sixth chakra (the third eye). This body enables you to receive insights and intuition. When this body is fully functioning, your spiritual purpose becomes clear. You are then able to use the physical body to manifest your spiritual purpose on earth.

7: Nirvanic Body

The nirvanic body is your Divine body, sometimes referred to as your light body. It has no boundaries so it is a massive body of light. It is the finest of all seven bodies and links to the crown chakra. When your crown chakra is open and balanced then your light body will be fully operational. This cannot happen until your other chakras have been brought into balance. This happens when you have cleared your sushumna enough to allow a large amount of chi/prana to flow through your system. At that stage you will be living for others rather than for yourself. You will have freed yourself from the hold of the ego and you will view everything as sacred. Sacred and Divine is not 'out there' or 'up there' but is right here.

Chapter 10

Questions and Answers

What happens if one of my chakras is completely blocked?

It is not possible for a chakra to be completely blocked. A chakra might only have a small amount of energy running through it but there will always be SOME energy there.

I have heard that there are more than seven chakras. Is that true?

Yes. In this book I have discussed the seven main chakras that are directly linked to the physical body, but there are many minor chakras such as those in the centre of our palms and at the back of the knees. There are also chakras above and below the physical body.

What are higher and lower chakras?

Of the seven chakras, the first three are called the lower chakras, the heart is the centre and the fifth, sixth and seventh are called the higher chakras.

What is prana?

Prana is the name of the life force energy that permeates everything in existence. Some people call it chi. It is prana that flows through our energy bodies and makes our chakras spin.

Is there a fast way of getting my chakras in balance?

Each of the chakras has 'seed syllables'. By chanting these sounds on a regular basis you can use the power of sound vibration to harmonise your chakras. Do this in conjunction with the 'How can I balance my chakra?' exercises listed under each chakra description. The solfeggio frequencies are also very powerful and effective. Reiki can assist in balancing and healing all the chakras.

What is the aura?

This is the energy field that surrounds the physical body. It is formed of coloured light. The brilliance, shade and size of the aura varies according to the state of the chakras.

Is there a guided meditation to heal all the chakras at once?

The Golden Shower.

Sit in a comfortable position on the floor or on a chair with the spine upright and the face and shoulders relaxed. Imagine that above you is a beam of golden light. As you breathe in visualise this light entering your body through the top of your head. As you exhale imagine this light travelling down your body, through your legs and out of your feet. The 'crossover' between the in and the out breath might occur in the area of the throat, the heart, the belly or elsewhere. There is no right or wrong crossover point. Whatever feels right for you IS right for you.

After a few minutes of using this breathing technique the beam of golden light becomes a shower. You are now sitting under a very large shower head with golden light pouring out instead of water. Your whole body is flooded with this light. Now you can just breathe normally, allowing your body to be soaked by the golden light.

After a few minutes sitting under this light shower, go back to using the breathing technique. As you breathe in, draw the shower of light through the top of your head right down to your feet, thereby filling your body with light. As you breathe out send the light out of your body in all directions. It fills the area around your body in the shape of an egg. With each breath you intensify the light that surrounds you. Sit within this golden egg for as long as you wish, knowing that by doing so you are cleansing your entire energy system.

When you are ready to finish, take a deep breath in through your nose, exhale slowly and completely through the mouth through pursed lips. Do this three times. Rub your hands vigorously together until they are hot, then place a hand on each cheek. Repeat the hand rubbing but this time place the hot hands on your abdomen. Finally repeat and place the hot hands on the soles of your feet.

I did the questionnaires in this book and all of my chakras are out of balance. Is that normal?

I would say that is not unusual. Some will be more unbalanced than others so I suggest you start by working on the most imbalanced ones first.

I did the questionnaires and all of my chakras are in perfect balance. Is that normal?

I would say that is unusual. However, if that is so then I suggest that you now work on increasing the amount of prana/chi/energy flowing through your chakras. To do this, alkalise your body, stretch your muscles, practise abdominal breathing, eat fresh and pure food, spend time in nature and be happy!

I am working on healing my chakras but my partner isn't. Does that matter?

We tend to draw towards us partners who mirror our unresolved issues. When you work on healing your chakras you begin to change as a person. If you change and your partner doesn't then you are likely to find that the relationship will either adjust or end.

Does the Earth have chakras?

Yes. Earth has seven continents and there is one chakra on each continent. They are thought to be as follows:

1st chakra – Mount Shasta, California
2nd chakra – Lake Titicaca, South America
3rd chakra – Uluru (Ayers Rock), Australia
4th chakra – Glastonbury-Shaftesbury, England
5th chakra – Great Pyramid, Giza, Egypt
6th chakra – Kuh-e Malek Siah, Iran
7th chakra – Mount Kailash, Tibet

What is kundalini?

Kundalini (koon-da-lee-nee) is coiled energy situated at the base of the spine. It is almost always taught that through yoga practises, the kundalini unwinds and travels up the sushumna. However, some yogis believe that what actually happens is that the kundalini, that 'sleeping serpent' at the base of the spine, is destroyed through correct yoga practises. Once it is out of the way, the energy/prana can then enter the sushumna and travel upwards, dramatically increasing the amount of energy flowing through your energy channels. The removal of the sleeping serpent is like a door opening.

What are the knots?

Within the sushumna channel are three psychic knots known as granthis. As kundalini energy rises it has to pierce these knots. Each time a knot is pierced, your consciousness is raised.

The three knots are:

Brahma. This is located in the first chakra.
Visnu. This is located at the fourth chakra.
Rudra. This is located in the sixth chakra. When the kundalini energy manages to pierce this knot, increased energy can flow to the crown chakra, greatly expanding the level of consciousness.

How do the glands affect the chakras?

Each chakra is loosely linked to a gland. You could think of these seven glands as seven people, each in charge of one gland and therefore one chakra. Each person is of equal importance. They communicate with each other through the bloodstream. They tell the other glands what state their health is in. They send their messages through hormones. The better they are able to communicate, the better your energy can flow.

What are nadis?

Nadi translates as 'flow'. Nadis are the fine energy channels. You will be familiar with your physical body and the way that the blood flows through major arteries and veins right down to the tiny capillaries. Energy flows in our energy body in a very similar way but through the nadis rather than through the blood vessels. There are thought to be 72,000 nadis. They carry prana, not blood. The three most important nadis are called ida, pingala and sushumna. All three run along the spine.

Why is Hatha Yoga called Hatha?

'Ha' means Ida Nadi. It flows through the left nostril. It is feminine, yin, cold and lunar.

'Tha' means Pingala Nadi. It flows through the right nostril. It is masculine, yang, hot and solar.

Hatha refers to the balance between Ida and Pingala.

The basic purpose of Hatha Yoga is to purify the Ida and Pingala Nadis and increase the amount of prana flowing through the sushumna. When the channels are clear the energy rises through the sushumna and the crown chakra can open fully.

Exercise

Lie down somewhere comfortable and breathe softly in and out through the nose. Bring your awareness to the top lip, just below your nostrils. Observe the breath entering and leaving your nose. Does one nostril feel more open than the other? Does it feel as if more air is entering through one nostril? Or do they feel exactly the same?

If your right nostril felt more active you are in a sun phase. You are currently activating your hot PINGALA channel. If it was the left nostril then you are in a moon phase. You are currently activating your cool IDA channel. Every two hours our breath changes from one nostril to the other and it is only when the transfer is taking place that the two nostrils take in an equal and balanced amount of air.

Sometimes you can become so off balance that one nostril remains dominant throughout the day and night, which can indicate physical, mental, or emotional difficulties.